Is
Clinton's
Health Care
Plan
Socialized
Medicine?

Is Clinton's Health Care Plan Socialized Medicine?

by Kimberly C. Parker

Huntington House Publishers

Huntington House Publishers
P.O. Box 53788
Lafayette, Louisiana 70505

Library of Congress
Card Catalog Number 94-76322
ISBN 1-56384-070-7

Contents

v

Introduction

Presidential candidate Bill Clinton made health care reform a central part of his campaign. He portrayed himself as a crusader for the middle class—a new Democrat—devoted to helping average Americans through tax cuts and reform of the health care system. But, election victory brought about a metamorphosis in this "new Democrat." Candidate Clinton's promises to the middle class were abandoned while President Clinton catered to the whims of liberal special interest groups.

Today, Mr. Clinton is engrossed in yet another campaign, the campaign for the Health Security Act. Again, he dons the image of crusader, campaigning for "compassionate solutions" to the average

American's health care concerns. But, our memories must not fail us. Mr. Clinton's first year in office proved where his heart lies, and it is not with middle class or average America. If there remains any doubt that Mr. Clinton is a liberal's liberal, a review of this legislation should convince even the most naive of Americans.

There is undoubtedly room for improvement in our nation's health care system, but the American public must realize that the provisions of the Clinton Health Security Act have much more to do with the president's espousal of a particular ideology and philosophy of government than they do with quality health care in America. Mr. Clinton is an advocate of strict federal government control who determined some time ago to begin his push toward socialism with the health care system.

Mr. Clinton promotes this legislation as a "compassionate" response to the "crisis" in health care, but the truth is that he created the "crisis" to justify his legislation. He misrepresented the figures on the number of uninsured Americans, lamented over the impending doom of rising health care costs, and established the unattainable goal of universal coverage as a moral imperative—all to justify the measures in this legislation that will rob us of individual freedoms and begin the drift toward complete government control of our economy.

The challenge before the American public is to look beyond the rhetoric in this debate to the facts. This handbook will endeavor to present the facts—facts about the fabricated health care crisis, facts about the Health Security Act and its hollow promises, and the facts about other countries' experiences with socialized medicine.

America was founded upon the principles of individual liberty and responsibility. The legislation we adopt to answer the problems in health care delivery must remain true to these fundamental principles. We cannot abandon the values we hold dear for hollow promises of "health security."

1

The "Crisis"

1. What are the accurate figures on the number of uninsured Americans in this country?

Current estimates indicate that at any one time thirty-nine million Americans are uninsured. However, statistics from the National Center for Policy Analysis (NCPA) demonstrate that this figure is misleading when presented as though these thirty-nine million Americans are permanently disenfranchised. Of the thirty-nine million, roughly half, or 19.5 million, will be insured in less than four months. Three-fourths will be insured in twelve months.

NCPA data indicates that only 2.5 percent of the population, or six million people, remain uninsured for more than two years. Profiles of these Americans indicate that most of them are young and healthy. Many have below-average incomes, but 3.8 million live in households with annual incomes of fifty thousand dollars or more. Three and one-half million have a bachelor's degree and one hundred thousand have a Ph.D. Roughly 2.7 million are self-employed.[1]

These figures tell a much different story than one imagines when hearing reports about the uninsured. Many of these people can afford health insurance but have chosen not to purchase it because they deem the costs too high relative to its benefits for this particular time in their lives.

2. Is the goal of universal coverage attainable?

Again, data from the NCPA indicates that the chronically uninsured include the long-term unemployed, drug dealers, prostitutes, and "others who work in the underground economy."[2] Many of these people are transient or unemployed and, therefore, beyond the reach of any government system when they so desire.

NCPA notes that any time you are requiring people to do something, and

particularly pay for something, there will
be those who avoid the system. One example is the fact that forty-one states and
the District of Columbia require motor-
ists to have liability insurance, yet estimates indicate that one in seven are not
insured. Coercion simply does not work
because the sanctions are difficult to
enforce.[3]

One final point that must be made is
that universal health coverage is only de-
sirable if it is voluntary. As Merrill
Matthews and Morgan Reynolds of NCPA
point out, the "federal government has
no constitutional authority to coerce
people into purchasing health
insurance"(Merrill Matthews and Morgan
O. Reynolds, "Some Questions We Ought
To Be Asking About Health Care," *The
Washington Times* [4 February 1984]:
A21). This legislation not only requires
that individuals be insured, but assesses
civil monetary penalties of up to five
thousand dollars, or three times the premiums (whichever is greater), for re-
peated failure to pay.[4]

**3. From the onset of this debate,
great alarm resounded over the fact
that health care costs continue to**

**consume a greater percentage of the
Gross Domestic Product (GDP). Has
the rise in health care costs created
a crisis, or is this alarmist rhetoric
just part and parcel of the Clinton
facade?**

William J. Baumol, director of the
C.V. Starr Center for Applied Econom-
ics at New York State University, ad-
dresses the rising costs of health care in
an issue of *The New Republic*. Dr. Baumol
explains this trend as a logical consequence of the differing rates of productivity between a labor-intensive industry
like health care and less labor-intensive
sectors of our economy (more detailed
explanation later). The rate of productivity (measure of the labor hours used to
produce one unit of a product) rises at a
slower pace in health care because service industries are labor intensive. Baumol
explains, "In an economy in which productivity is growing in almost every sector and declining in none, . . . consumers can have more of every good and
service; they simply have to transfer some
of the gains from the sector that's becoming much more productive into the

sector that's becoming only a little more productive."[5]

The problem with focusing on the growing percentage of the pie is that it obscures the fact that the entire pie is growing—growth made possible by the increases in productivity in the less labor-intensive sectors of the economy. The sectors where productivity is increasing more rapidly allow us to afford more and better health care as well as many other things.[6]

4. What about the future? Can this trend continue?

According to Baumol's analysis, this trend can continue.

> Imagine that the real price of health care continues to rise at its current rate for fifty years, and that overall U.S. productivity rises for that period at its historic rate of around 2 percent. In fifty years, the output of every good and service, including education and health care, can increase to more than 3.5 times its 1990 magnitude: an enormous increase in wealth for everyone. But the relative composition of the sectors will be drastically different.

Medical outlays, instead of constituting 12 percent of the total, as they did in 1990, would rise to more than 35 percent in 2040 (Baumol, "Do Health Care Costs Matter?" *The New Republic* [22 November 1933]: 18).

5. Does the fact that our society can afford to spend more on health care mean we should not be concerned about the rise in costs?

No. Our nation can do a better job of controlling the rise in health care costs. There are certain aspects of our health care system that encourage waste. The fact that third parties (insurance companies) pay the bulk of medical expenses leads to increased costs because neither physician nor patient have any incentive to be cost-conscious.

Another area in need of reform is medical liability. Malpractice suits account for about 5 percent of physicians' revenues and contribute to the number of procedures that physicians require. According to the consulting firm Lewin-VHI, defensive medicine—tests or procedures that doctors require to prevent malpractice suits—account for about $25 million in costs annually.[7]

Just because our nation can afford to pay rising medical costs does not mean that we should not be cost-conscious or rectify unnecessary trends that lead to waste. On the contrary, we should do everything we can to keep costs down. The important thing to remember, however, is that health care spending is not the "crisis" the Clinton administration claims it to be.

2 | The Health Security Act

The Health Security Act proposes complete government control of the health care system. No aspect of health care delivery escapes the reach of this 1,364 page document. Robert Moffet, deputy director of Domestic and Economic Policy Studies at the Heritage Foundation describes the act as a "massive top-down, bureaucratic command-and-control system"(Robert E. Moffett, "A Guide to the Clinton Health Plan," *Heritage Talking Points*, [19 November 1993]: 1). It is indeed no exaggeration to state that the passage of this legislation will effectively socialize one- seventh of our nation's economy.

The act creates an independent National Health Board that divides responsibility with existing executive agencies for the administration of the health care system at the national level. It sets national standards and oversees the establishment and administration of the health care system by the states.

The National Health Board is a seven-member, presidentially-appointed entity with the power to "establish such rules as may be necessary to carry out this Act."[1] Its responsibilities include supervision of the state system, management of the comprehensive benefit package, oversight and enforcement of a national budget, quality management and supervision of breakthrough drug prices. It also has the power to establish standards regarding medical necessity—standards that could jeopardize the health and well-being of many Americans.

The states are charged with implementing and enforcing federal health care policy. Each must designate an agency or official to coordinate state responsibilities under federal law. States must establish one or more regional health alliances, with one, and only one, alliance serving each geographic area. States are also required to enforce budgeting and spending levels.

These regional "monopolies" can operate as non profit corporations, independent state agencies, or an agency of the state executive branch. Each alliance must negotiate and contract with at least three state-certified health plans that provide, at a minimum, the standard benefit package; enroll employers and employees; manage access to plans; collect premiums; and pay the plans, which, in turn, reimburse providers.

Companies with five thousand or more employees can establish a corporate alliance, supervised by the Department of Labor. Corporate alliances operate under much the same regulations as regional alliances.

The legislation outlines a "comprehensive benefit package" that must be available to every individual at the same premium regardless of risk. Eighteen categories of treatments are spelled out over fifty-six pages, and delivery of these services is required of any health plan that wishes to be state-certified. No regional alliance may carry a plan that is not approved by the state.

The benefit package includes everything from hospital services to outpatient

prescription drugs to vision and dental
care. The government-mandated package
also includes family planning services and
services for pregnant women, including
abortion.

The system is largely financed by employers and employees, with employers
picking up the greater part of the tab.
Employers will be required to offer the
standard benefit package to their employees and pay at least 80 percent of the
cost of the average plan. Employees will
pay the remaining amount of the premiums. No employer in any regional alliance will be required to pay more than
7.9 percent of payroll annually for health
coverage.

While the administration claims that
a national health care budget will only
serve as a "backstop" to organized market power, what one envisions in the
pages of this legislation is anything but a
free market at work. One of the primary
responsibilities of the National Health
Board is to issue regulations concerning
the implementation and enforcement of
a national budget. The board decides how
much a nation can spend and imposes
premium targets and caps on the growth
in premiums to keep costs within bud-

get. Each state is charged with enforcing the global budget imposed on it by the National Health Board.

While the president continues to refer to his proposal as one of "managed competition," it strays from the concept of managed competition in that it adds global budgeting and price controls. Premium caps serve as the mechanism to lower costs, eventually requiring that premiums rise at the rate of general inflation, a rate well below that of health care cost inflation. Prospective budgeting and fee schedules are imposed upon so-called fee-for-service plans.

1. Am I assured access to every item or service in the "comprehensive benefit package"?

The legislation states that the "comprehensive benefit package" does not include an "item or service that the National Health Board may determine is not medically necessary or appropriate."[2] The board is charged with establishing the regulations necessary to determine "medical necessity" or "appropriateness."[3]

Given these provisions, the fact that a service is listed in the benefit package does not necessarily guarantee a patient access to that service under this legislation. The patient's access to the service is determined by regulations from the National Health Board.

2. Can I choose not to enroll in a regional alliance?

No. An individual must enroll in a plan or the alliance assigns them to the lowest-cost plan available. The penalty for not enrolling in an applicable health plan in a timely fashion is "payment of twice the amount of the family share of premiums."[4]

There are people who choose not to carry health insurance for personal reasons. For example, the *Christian Brotherhood Newsletter,* based in Barberton, Ohio, coordinates the payment of medical bills through voluntary contributions from subscriber to subscriber. The group has paid the medical bills of over thirty thousand people since 1982. Last year alone, newsletter subscribers paid more than $27 million in medical expenses. Under the Clinton plan, the *Christian Brotherhood* subscribers would not have the freedom to opt out of an alliance.

3. Can a geographic area offer more than one alliance to promote competition within the region?

The legislation specifically states, "No geographic area may be assigned to more than one regional alliance."[5]

4. Do states have the option of choosing a different type of system than the alliance system imposed by this legislation?

The only alternative to the regional alliance "monopolies" is a single-payer system, which creates a state monopoly. The single-payer system tightens government control and offers only one state-prescribed health plan, which provides at least the minimum "comprehensive benefit package."[6] This legislation actually encourages states to establish heavy-handed single-payer systems by relieving them of certain requirements imposed upon the alliances.

In a single-payer system, the states must, "in a manner satisfactory to the Board," ensure that they stay within budget just as if the state were a single regional alliance. "Automatic, mandatory, nondiscretionary reduction in payments

, health care providers" are expected if paying these providers would force the state to exceed its budget.[7]

5. Am I assured of having the option of a fee-for-service (choose-your-own-doctor) health plan?

No. Although the legislation does require that each alliance offer at least one so-called fee-for-service plan, the provision is disingenuous for several reasons.

First, the legislation states that an alliance cannot offer a contract to a plan in which the proposed premium exceeds the weighted-average premium within the alliance by more than 20 percent. Most fee-for-service plans could not compete under this provision.[8]

Secondly, the bill calls for the regional alliance or state to develop a "prospective budget" for providers in fee-for-service plans. The negotiated budget establishes spending targets for the plan and each sector or field of medicine. The legislation requires that if the regional alliance or state determines that using these services may cause it to exceed its budget(s), the "plan shall reduce the amount of payments otherwise made to providers (through a withhold or delay in payments or adjustments) in such manner and by such amounts as necessary to assure that expenditures will not exceed the budget."[9] These provisions will make it difficult for fee-for-service plans to compete.

Thirdly, the plans are not pure fee-for-service plans where patients select their physicians and physicians are free to practice according to their conscience and their best medical knowledge. Fee schedules will be established to govern reimbursement, limiting what health plans can pay doctors and prohibiting patients from supplementing the amount specified. These fee-for-service plans are also subject to "reasonable requirements," which may include utilization review (review of doctor's recommendations by a designated entity) or prior approval for certain services.[10] Fee schedules and "reasonable requirements" will prevent physicians from practicing according to their conscience or in the best interest of their patient. Many physicians in independent practice will be forced into "managed care" plans due to their inability to compete within the schedules.

This legislation in effect pushes people into Health Maintenance Organi-

zations (HMOs) or their less restrictive
cousin Preferred Physician Organizations
(PPOs). As Mahattan Institute Fellow
Elizabeth McCaughey notes, "The bill is
designed to push people into HMOs
(Health Maintenance Organizations)
which restrict your choice of physicians
and hospitals, and use gatekeepers to
curb the use of specialists, expensive tests,
and costly high tech treatments."[11]

6. Are there any alternatives to the regional health alliances?

Only one. Firms with five thousand
or more employees nationwide may elect
to establish a "corporate alliance" rather
than enroll in a regional health alliance.
These corporate alliances are for the most
part subject to the same federal and state
requirements and must offer at least the
standard benefit package. The secretary
of labor is charged with the oversight of
these alliances.

There are several significant disincen-
tives for large employers considering the
formation of a corporate alliance. One is
that the firm, rather than the federal government, is required to subsidize the premium payments of low-wage, full-time

workers.[12] Corporate alliance employers are also required to pay an additional 1 percent payroll tax.[13] A third disincentive is that the secretary of labor has the authority to impose an "assessment" of up to 2 percent on the insurance premiums of corporate alliances to finance the Corporate Alliance Health Plan Insolvency Fund.[14]

7. Do corporate alliances have to offer the same choice of plans?

Yes. A corporate alliance must offer the choice of at least three plans including one fee-for-service plan. Again, citizens must recognize that a true fee-for-service plan will not exist under this legislation and some experts say the "choice" will "vanish" altogether.

8. President Clinton campaigned on the promise of introducing the concept of "managed competition" into America's health care system? What is managed competition?

According to the National Center for Policy Analysis (NCPA), advocates of "managed competition" believe that this concept is a "workable middleground"

between the "polar extremes of socialized medicine and free markets."[15] In
"managed competition," employees
choose from a variety of health insurance plans with the employer paying a
fixed sum and the employee paying the
remainder of the premium. Premiums are
fixed on the basis of "community rating"
or charging the same amount to every
individual in the plan regardless of the
cost or risk the individual brings to the
plan.

Under managed competition, insurers are no longer competing on the basis
of their ability to price and manage risk.
Instead, insurers become managers of
health care delivery, and they compete
on their ability to manage cost.

9. Does managed competition work?

Managed competition cannot work
because it creates an artificial health insurance market based upon premiums
that have nothing to do with the value of
the insurance people receive. In a com-
petitive market, the prices of premiums
are based upon the risk or cost a person
brings to the pool. Thus, market forces
dictate that the price of the premium
tends to be equal to the insurance re-
ceived.

Under managed competition, the premium for every individual is set and only varies with family size, not health risk. A person with AIDS would pay the same premium as a healthy individual even though the individual with AIDS brings much greater risk and cost to the pool. Thus, insurers are no longer managers of risk (because they cannot adjust price based upon risk), but are nothing more than managers of health care delivery. The only way to effectively manage delivery under community rating is to manage cost.

The management of cost rather than risk creates perverse incentives for insurers that cause serious problems in health care delivery. First, managed competition changes the health care market. Insurers are no longer selling insurance against risky events. Premiums are prepayment for the consumption of medical services, and this change in premiums alters the way insurers compete.

Plans attempt to avoid the sickest and most in need of services. In order to manage cost, they cater to the needs of healthy individuals, not those in the greatest need of care. They tend to provide more pre-

ventive care—care that healthy individuals can use—rather than concentrating on
services for chronic conditions that might
attract individuals who would drive up
costs.

Secondly, plans are forced to
underprovide to the sick and overprovide
to the healthy. With community rating,
the sick tend to pay much less in premiums than they cost a plan, so services
and technology for the sickest patients
are cut in order to adjust cost down to
the premium paid. Likewise, healthy
individuals are forced to overpay so costs
have to be adjusted up to the premium
level by offering the healthy more services.

Thirdly, fee-for-service plans are
pushed out of the market because they
cannot compete with "managed care"
plans. Independent practitioners who stay
in private practice so they can treat patients as they see fit cannot compete with
"managed care" plans that operate based
upon projected cost.

Fourth, there is no incentive for plans
to invest money in innovative treatments
for chronic illnesses or disease. Since
plans do not want to attract the sick, they

have no motivation for researching and developing new methods of treatment for serious illnesses.

Finally, the quality of health care delivery in general will suffer while premiums will rise for most people. With cost as the bottom line, physicians will tend to offer only the minimal service. Every individual will receive less care, and most will pay more for it. Note that "community rating" places an undue burden on healthy individuals in mandating that they subsidize (through increased premiums) the risky lifestyles of others.[16]

10. Does "managed competition" decrease costs?

Most research indicates that if managed competition decreases cost, it is a one-time shot in the arm. Some studies indicate that managed care techniques can lead to one-time reductions of as much as 10 to 15 percent by substituting less expensive therapies. However, because managed care plans make services "free" at the time of consumption, many patients tend to overconsume, offsetting the one-time reductions.[17]

11. Is the Clinton proposal based

upon the concept of "managed competition?"

Yes, but it will wreak greater havoc because it combines the concept of "managed competition" with global budgeting and price controls. As already mentioned, managed competition creates the tendency to sacrifice quality in the delivery of services because it is the only way for plans to compete. Global budgeting and price controls only make these problems worse.

Rationing is a much greater risk under the Clinton proposal because it sets a standard benefit package that all plans must provide. Setting premium ceilings and a floor on benefits means that the only way plans can compete is to ration services to certain segments of the population, ration on the basis of regulations regarding "medical necessity" and "appropriateness," and/or reduce the quality of care through waiting lists and limited access to advanced technology.

12. Will my family be able to purchase the care we need if the "comprehensive benefit package" proves inadequate or in the event that treatment is considered "inappropriate?"

The legislation specifically states, "No health plan, insurer, or any other person may offer to any eligible individual a supplemental health benefit policy that duplicates any coverage provided in the comprehensive benefit package."[18] Even if the services provided in the "comprehensive benefit package" are inadequate, an individual will probably not be able to buy more insurance to meet their needs. Individuals can only obtain additional services by paying directly for them. Section 1003 of Title I states, "Nothing in this Act shall be construed as prohibiting an individual from purchasing any health care services."[19] Note that this provision does not mean the purchase of insurance. It means direct out-of-pocket payments in after-tax dollars.

It is also important to note again that this plan discourages physicians from remaining in private practice; "managed care" plans may regulate what their providers can do on a fee-for-service basis. So, even if an individual has the money to pay for services out-of-pocket, physicians who perform the service may be in short supply.

13. What types of services can be

covered under the supplemental insurance plans?

Services like cosmetic surgery or long-term rehabilitative treatment may be covered by supplemental insurance packages.

14. Will part-time workers be covered under the Clinton plan?

Yes, employers will be required to pay a portion of part-time workers premiums, but the amount will be pro rated on the basis of the hours worked by that employee.

15. How will Medicare be affected?

The act does not require the dissolution of Medicare, but the language does authorize states, if they so desire, to abolish Medicare within their boundaries. If states choose this option, they must fold the recipients into the alliance system and assure that beneficiaries have access to the same or better coverage, and federal liability is not increased.[20]

If a state chooses not to act upon this authorization, Medicare recipients retain the option to remain under Medicare or join the alliance system.

This act does call for significant cuts

in Medicare spending to control costs. Burke J. Balch of the National Right to Life Committee reports that cuts could add up to roughly $124 billion.[21]

No later than 1 July 1996, a new prescription drug benefit is added to the Medicare package. The benefit carries with it a $250 annual deductible. Once the deductible has been met, beneficiaries pay only 20 percent of the cost of each prescription with an annual out-of-pocket limit on expenditures of one thousand dollars.[22]

One cost-cutting measure proposed in this act will seriously compromise the ability of Medicare beneficiaries to obtain the prescription drugs they need. The secretary of HHS is given the authority to set a controlled price on drugs and require drug manufacturers to pay a rebate on each unit sold to Medicare patients. If the manufacturers refuse to pay the rebate, the secretary has the authority to blacklist the drugs, striking them from the list of prescriptions eligible for Medicare reimbursement. This measure is yet another indication that the well-being of individuals will run a distant second to the priority of controlling costs.[23]

16. What about Medicaid recipients?

Medicaid recipients will be fully integrated into regional alliance system with their premiums subsidized by the federal government.

17. In urban areas with high concentrations of Medicaid recipients, will folding these people into the alliances affect premiums?

Yes, urban alliances will pay the highest price for mainstreaming Medicaid recipients into the alliance system. Every individual in those urban alliances will pay more in order to offset the shifts in cost from Medicaid to local premiums.

18. Are federal government employees required to join the regional alliance system?

The Department of Defense will establish its own health care system as will the Veterans Administration and the Indian Health Service. These systems will operate outside the state regional alliances.

Federal employees covered by the Federal Employee Health Benefits Program (FEHBP) will join the regional alliances, but only after the rest of the eligible Americans have joined the system. The FEHBP is to be abolished effective 31 December 1997.

19. Does the Clinton proposal increase or decrease the bureaucracy of the health care system?

The Clinton act adds numerous new levels of bureaucracy to a system already hampered by red tape. It would create twenty-five new entities and/or programs under the National Health Board, seventy-eight new entities and/or programs from the departments of the executive branch to individuals and families. While President Clinton claims that this proposal will reduce paperwork, the sea of paper this bureaucracy would create is staggering to contemplate. The time lags generated by this system will unquestionably compromise the efficient delivery of services.

20. Privacy is so important in the doctor-patient relationship. Will this

**legislation compromise the confiden-
tiality of this relationship?**

An intricate information network is
established under the Clinton plan to
monitor compliance with government
regulation. This proposal is staggering in
its attempts to micromanage a system of
this size and magnitude. Every visit to a
system is logged into a national data bank
and reviewed by examiners. Privacy is
compromised to ensure compliance.

21. How does the Clinton adminis-
tration propose to finance this "command-and-control" health care system?

Mr. Clinton proposes a combination
of employer/employee financing, shifts
of funding from federal programs like
Medicare, Medicaid, and other government health programs, along with some
new taxes and projected tax revenues.

Employers contributions pay for 80
percent of the average priced plan offered in the alliance for each family type
with employees paying the difference. No
employer (except corporate alliance employers) is required to pay more than 7.9
percent of payroll for health coverage an-

nually. Firms with fewer than fifty employees are eligible for limits from 3.5 to 7.9 percent of payroll.

The federal government will subsidize the premium payments of families and individuals in regional alliances whose income is below 150 percent of poverty. Low-wage workers in corporate alliances will be subsidized by the employer.

According to the testimony of Donna Shalala, additional financing for the plan will come from cuts in Medicare, Medicaid, and federal employee health benefits totaling $230 billion; another $89 billion from a sin tax on tobacco and a corporate tax on those firms opting out of the alliance system; and finally $71 billion from tax revenues on projected wage and profit increases.[24]

Despite claims by the Clinton administration that the plan will be fully funded and even decrease the deficit by $58 billion, many economists are concerned that costs will completely outstrip funding and significantly increase the deficit. The federal government is notorious for underestimating the costs and projected annual increases of new entitlement programs. When Medicare was created in the 1960s, budget projections estimated that it would reach 9 to 12 billion by 1990. The actual cost in 1990 was 107 billion.

Many economists have reviewed the Clinton estimates to cover the comprehensive benefit package, concluding that the administration's estimates are too low. The White House claims that the package will cost individuals $1,932, and families $4,360. Two private studies have estimated the cost of the benefit package for families at $5,900 and $6,662 respectively.[25] Congressional Budget Office (CBO) projections are that health care premiums will be about 15 percent higher than administration estimates.[26]

Thirdly, White House projections were that the plan would produce $290 billion in savings between 1995 to 2000 while the CBO arrived at quite different figures. CBO director Robert Reischauer estimated that the plan will boost the size of the federal government by 20 percent while increasing federal spending by $56 billion in 1996 and more than $700 billion by 2004. He also stated that it would increase the federal deficit by $74 billion despite the Clinton administration's claim of a $58 billion reduction. CBO projects the higher deficit because it believes the Clinton administration underestimated the amount the federal government will have to pay businesses to subsidize the cost of health insurance.[27]

22. If employers are required to provide their employees insurance and pay 80 percent of the cost, can we expect job losses?

The primary author of the Clinton plan, Ira Magaziner, contends that this legislation will create jobs, but most liberal and conservative economists disagree, expecting unemployment to grow as a result of employer mandates. Professors June and David O'Neill of Baruch College for the Washington-based Employment Policies Institute estimate job loss at 3.1 million. The Employee Benefit Research Institute estimates that as many as 1.2 million workers could lose their jobs. Even the president's economic advisers estimate that about six hundred thousand jobs could be lost.[28]

23. Will our taxes increase as a result of this proposal?

In all likelihood, yes. Private consulting firms as well as the Congressional Budget Office (CBO) think that the Clinton administration has underestimated the cost of the proposal and overestimated the ability of proposed fiscal constraints to control cost. Furthermore, if the substance of this legislation passes, government control will inevitably expand and costs with it. If the administration has indeed underestimated the cost of this huge entitlement program, the alternative to reducing care is a robust tax increase.

24. What other economic consequences can we expect from this employer mandate?

Employer mandates on insurance affect labor costs. When labor costs rise, businesses pass on the burden of those increased costs. Employees who retain their jobs may suffer wage reductions and fewer non health benefits. Consumers will share the burden through increased prices.

25. How will medical schools be affected?

This legislation requires that a National Council on Graduate Medical Education be established within the Department of Health and Human Services. This council will designate for each academic year the number of individuals authorized to be enrolled in eligible specialty programs. After a five-year phase in period, the number of physicians trained in primary care must be at least 55 percent of the total with percentage increases each year for primary care and percentage decreases in specialty care in fields where the council determines excess supply exists. Primary care includes family medicine, general internal medicine, and general pediatrics.

In a purported attempt to bring primary care and specialty care into balance, this legislation would drastically reduce the number of specialists available to treat serious conditions. Not only will it be hard to see a specialist, but there will be fewer and fewer physicians with the necessary training to research and develop new treatment methods.[29]

26. Does the Clinton proposal offer any serious medical liability reform?

The Clinton proposal's medical liability reform provisions are weak. It offers an "Alternative Dispute Resolution System," but neither this system nor the other provisions offer any meaningful solutions.

3

The Impact upon Our Children

As mentioned earlier, this legislation is about the promotion of a particular ideology, and nothing demonstrates that more clearly than the provisions which deal with family planning and pregnancy-related services, school-based health clinics, and comprehensive health education. The provisions regarding these three aspects of (dis)service reveal, beyond a shadow of a doubt, that Mr. Clinton is attempting to use the health care package and the command-and-control system it creates to accomplish what he and his cohorts have been unable to accomplish in the federal and state legislatures.

1. Does the "comprehensive benefit package" cover abortion?

Yes! The "comprehensive benefit package" guarantees access to family planning services and pregnancy related services.[1] President Clinton stated on MTV that abortion is included in pregnancy related services; Mrs. Clinton testified to the same before the Senate Finance Committee, and Donna Shalala, in a speech to the National Abortion and Reproductive Rights Action League (NARAL), added her assurance that women would have "full reproductive rights" under the Clinton plan. In essence, passage of this legislation will ensure that abortion becomes a federally guaranteed benefit. It is indeed a gross perversion of authority for our federal government to give abortion the status of a routine medical procedure under the guise of promoting our nation's "health"!

Pro life Representative Henry Hyde (R-IL) stated in testimony before the Health Subcommittee of the House Energy and Commerce Committee,

> I can say, without exaggeration, that President Clinton's health care bill contains the most extreme pro-abortion provisions of any legislation ever introduced in Congress . . . even more extreme than the Free-

dom of Choice Act. This bill repre-
sents an attempt to impose on the
entire population, by force of law,
the ideological position of a small
minority—that abortion must be
treated as indistinguishable from
any routine medical procedure.

Pro abortion advocates see the inclusion of abortion in the comprehensive
benefit package as a fundamental victory
and vow to do whatever it takes to keep
it in the act. At NARAL's Leadership
Summit on 7 January 1994, President
Kate Michelman told participants,

This battle for comprehensive
health care and national health care
is going to be a defining moment
for us in our efforts to ensure reproductive health and freedom of
choice. If we lose, the implications
are enormous and I want you to
leave this day and this weekend
absolutely devoted to organizing fu-
riously across this country on be-
half of this health care plan.

In a speech on 12 July 1993, Pamela
Maraldo, president of Planned Parenthood Federation of America stated, "We
must secure access to those [abortion]
rights in mainstream health care deliv-

ery, and once and for all put the abortion debate to rest."

2. Will my insurance premiums go toward financing abortion?

In paying into premium pools, all employees and employers will fund the abortions provided by the physicians in those pools. Coercing Americans to pay premiums into health plans that provide abortions as part of the government-mandated benefit package amounts to an assault on the consciences of millions of Americans to satisfy the whims of special interests who value convenience over unborn life.

Representative Chris Smith (R-NJ) stated, "The Clinton proposal will force every American—every taxpayer, every employer, every working woman, and every working man to be a party to the chemical poisoning or dismemberment of innocent children. Under the Clinton plan, an unborn child at any age of gestation will be vulnerable to the abuse of abortion."*

---

* Testimony before the Health Subcommittee of the House Energy and Commerce Committee, 26 January 1984 as reported in *NRL News* 3 February 1994.

This action was taken by the Clinton administration despite the fact that surveys demonstrate widespread disagreement with the inclusion of abortion coverage in any health plan. A CBS/*New York Times* poll in March 1993 specifically asked if abortion should be included in the basic plan and found that 72 percent opposed coverage.[2]

Two polls taken by the *New York Times* in March and June of 1993 found large majorities of women, the constituency these pro abortion groups claim to represent, opposed to including abortion in the benefit package. March results revealed a 73 percent majority, while the June poll found 65 percent opposed to its inclusion.[3]

3. How about my tax dollars? Will they also be used to pay for abortions under the Clinton plan?

Yes! The Clinton proposal calls for the federal government to subsidize the premium payments of low-income workers in the regional alliances. Thus, our tax dollars will be part of the premium pool of every plan—the pool drawn from to pay abortion providers.

Secondly, the Clinton proposal provides for Medicaid recipients to be included in the regional alliances of a state and offered the same basic benefit package at taxpayer expense. These measures would effectively nullify the Hyde Amendment, which prohibits the use of taxpayer dollars for abortion except in cases of rape, incest, or where the life of the mother is threatened.

4. Will individuals have the option of joining a plan that does not provide abortion?

No! Initially, President Clinton claimed that Americans would be offered a choice in plans that excluded abortion coverage. However, as with so many of Mr. Clinton's promises, this choice never materialized. The legislation clearly states that a plan cannot be state-certified if it does not provide all the services outlined in the "comprehensive benefit package." Regional alliances are prohibited from offering a plan that is not state-certified.

5. Will the fact that this bill makes abortion a guaranteed health benefit

expand the availability of the procedure?

When questioned, the First Lady claims that the administration seeks no change in access to abortion. Mrs. Clinton stated in a Cable News Network interview, "We are not increasing the availability or decreasing the availability of abortion. We are really trying to strike a balance so that we provide what is available now."[4]

Despite the First Lady's claims, her allies on the issue see this legislation as a vehicle for significant change in the status of abortion. Pamela Maraldo, president of Planned Parenthood Federation of America stated, "The inclusion of reproductive health services in a basic benefit package will truly constitute a 'defining moment' for reproductive rights in America."[5]

Estelle Rogers of the ACLU suggested that "putting abortion on an equal footing with other reproductive health services" could expand the number of abortion providers.[6]

The administration defends its inclusion of abortion in the basic package of benefits with claims that most private insurance plans cover abortion. However, they provide no evidence to support this assertion. The *St. Louis Post-Dispatch* reported on 24 September 1993 that "a spokesman for A. Foster Higgins, Inc., a national employee benefits consultant that surveys 2,500 employers a year, said such coverage is common in Health Maintenance Organizations, but unusual in fee-for-service plans and employers self-funded plans. Self-funded plans provide health coverage for 65 percent of American workers."[7]

Secondly, in order to be approved by regional alliances, health plans will have to make abortion services available and accessible to women. The Alan Guttmacher Institute reports that 83 percent of the counties in America have no abortion provider. Thus, health plans will see to it that abortion facilities spring up in communities all over this nation where clinics do not currently exist.

It is important to note that just the revocation of the Hyde Amendment and extending coverage to women on Medicaid would result in substantial increases in the number of abortions.

Wanda Franz, president of the National Right to Life Committee (NRLC) commented, "President Clinton is really proposing to employ the power of federal law to require all Americans to pay for abortion as a method of birth control. If he succeeds, the number of abortions will skyrocket" (Douglas Johnson, "White House Seeks to Conceal Plan to Compel Americans to Buy Mandatory Abortion-On-Demand Insurance," *NRL News*, [14 September 1993]: 1).

6. Are doctors and hospitals required to perform abortions?

The legislation includes a "conscience clause" which states, "A health professional or a health facility may not be required to provide an item or service in the comprehensive benefit package if the professional or facility objects to doing so on the basis of a religious belief or moral conviction."[8] This language only relieves them of obligation with respect to the provision of services. It does not protect doctors and/or hospitals as employers. As employers, they would still be required to contribute to the provision of abortion services through the premium pools and tax subsidies.

In testimony before a House committee, Mrs. Clinton also went to great lengths to explain that health alliances could not invoke the "conscience clause" to restrict abortion in a particular region.

7. What about churches?

As Ben Mitchell, director of Biomedical and Life Issues for the Christian Life Commission of the Southern Baptist Convention testified before a House committee, "By making abortion a requirement of the comprehensive benefit package, health care reform of the President's variety would compel every denomination and local congregation either to fund abortion or else break the law and suffer the penalties. Every congregation as an employer would be coerced to take money from the offering plate and offer it up to abortionists."*

---

* Testimony before the Health Subcommittee of the House Energy and Commerce Committee, 26 January 1984 as reported in *NRL News* 3 February 1994.

8. Are school-based health clinics (SBCs) included in the Clinton plan?

School-based health clinics are included in the Clinton proposal. In fact, the legislation calls for over $1 billion from 1996 to 2000 to be appropriated for the implementation of "school-related health services." State agencies or local community partnerships (when states do not apply) are encouraged to establish school health service sites.[9]

Although these clinics are presented as providers of routine medical services, the five hundred existing SBCs are the primary vehicles of abortion counseling and referral for our nation's teenagers. These clinics employ school authority to funnel teens into abortion facilities without the knowledge or consent of parents.

Monies will be allocated first to those communities that show "the most substantial level of need for such services" among ten to nineteen-year-olds "as measured by indicators of community health includ-ing . . . high rates of indicators of health risk among children and youth including . . . adolescent pregnancy, sexually transmitted disease. . . ."[10] With teen pregnancy mentioned as a health risk in-

dicator, there is every reason to believe
that contraceptive distribution and abortion counseling and referral will be an
integral part of the services provided in
these clinics.

The legislation also gives SBCs a special status as "essential community providers." During the first five years of reform, health plans are required to contract with and reimburse "essential community providers" to ensure continuity
of service.[11] Most providers have to apply
for this status, but SBCs as well as family
planning clinics receive automatic certifi-
cation.

The Clinton proposal also calls for
"investments in new health programs
such as SBCs to expand access to care
for under-served populations," "training
for school-based health providers," and
"outreach in support of family planning
services" (i.e., abortion counseling and
referral services).

9. Does the Clinton plan weigh in on the sex education debate?

The plan, in effect, federalizes "the
provision in kindergarten through grade

12 of sequential, age-appropriate, comprehensive health education programs." It provides for $50 million for each fiscal year (1995–2000) to "establish a national framework within which States can create comprehensive school health programs that target the health risk behaviors accounting for the majority of the morbidity and mortality among youth and adults, including . . . unintended pregnancy. . . ."[12]

In order to qualify, the program must be kindergarten through twelfth grade, and it must include components such as family life (a more palatable term for comprehensive sexuality education), growth and development, and prevention and control of disease. Grants are also available under this subtitle to "work with State and local health agencies and State and local educational agencies to reduce barriers to the implementation of comprehensive school health education programs in schools."[13]

4 | The Rationing of Health Care

While this legislation purports to offer "health security" to every American, provisions within the proposal effectively compromise this objective. Careful scrutiny of the proposal reveals that the Clintons are much more interested in government control than quality health care for the average American.

1. With the introduction of the Health Security Act, much discussion ensued on the fact that this plan will result in the rationing of health care services. What in the act leads to rationing?

As mentioned earlier, the Clinton proposal combines "managed competition" with global budgets and price controls.

The National Health Board sets a budget to determine how much our nation can spend on health care each year. Based on that budget, the board implements price controls on premiums to limit the amount of money paid into the system. The rise in premiums in regional alliances will be limited through a national inflation factor.

The inflation factor employed by this legislation is the Consumer Price Index (the measure of general inflation). After a brief transition period, the growth in premiums will be restricted to the level of the CPI. The problem lies in the fact that the rate of health care cost inflation is significantly higher than the rate of general inflation. For example, in the twelve months ending in November 1993, the rate of health care cost inflation was 5.5 percent compared with the 2.7 percent rate of general inflation for roughly the same period.

Beginning in 1999, the Clinton plan requires that premiums increase at no more than the CPI or the general rate of inflation and then a combination of that index and the growth in per capita real Gross Domestic Product (GDP). The administration claims that these caps will wring out waste from the system, and, for a period of time, they may do just that. However, the time will soon come when capping premiums at a rate far below health care cost inflation will result in rationing. According to Henry Aaron of the Brookings Institution, "most savings would come from changes in medical practice. Physicians would have to administer fewer tests, hospitalize less often, do less surgery and prescribe fewer medications."[1] Health insurance plans that must restrict premiums to the rise in general inflation will have no choice but to ration care as costs exceed the money in the system.

The legislation makes it easy for health plans to ration care. It states that denial can be based on a "determination that the treatment is not medically necessary or appropriate or is inconsistent with the plan's practice guidelines."[2]

The drafters of this legislation must know that rationing will occur because they make it a federal crime to give or receive a bribe for health care services in violation of this act. Conviction under this section carries with it fines and prison terms of up to fifteen years in a federal penitentiary.[3]

2. Why is the rate of health care cost inflation twice as high as the rate of general inflation?

The primary reason lies in the productivity of health care in relation to other sectors of the economy. Dr. William Baumol explains that the difference in the productivity of health care, a labor-intensive industry, and other more mechanized sectors of our economy accounts for the higher rate of health care costs. According to Baumol, "productivity means, by definition, that it requires ever less labor time to produce a unit of . . . a service" (Baumol, "Do Health Care Costs Matter?" *The New Republic,* [22 November 1933], 18). In more machine-oriented sectors of the economy, advances in technology replace labor hours and therefore increase productivity. However, in health care, technological advances do not have the same effect. In service industries like health care, advances in technology enhance labor's effectiveness, but they do not cut down on the number of labor hours. Even the most advanced technology requires constant supervision by health care professionals. Doctors must order tests, skilled technicians must run the machines, and specialists interpret the results.

Baumol explains that increases in productivity in health care tend to manifest themselves not in fewer labor hours, but in greater effectiveness, i.e., more efficient diagnoses, better treatments, greater cure rates. Thus, the productivity of health care in relation to other sectors of the economy will inevitably lag behind due to its labor-intensive nature.

Since providers are incurring greater costs than industries with rapidly rising productivity, they pass these rising costs on in the form of price increases at a higher rate.[4]

3. What will be the criteria for rationing care?

The Clintons know that rationing will occur and have already decided that the denial of treatment will be based upon a subjective "quality of life" criteria. First, as previously discussed, the legislation includes provisions for the National Health Board to decide what is "medically necessary" and/or "appropriate." Secondly, Mrs. Clinton testified before the Senate Finance Committee on 30 September

1993 that people "will know that they are not being denied treatment for any reason other than it is not appropriate—will not enhance the quality of life." Likewise, the president stated in a "Meet the Press" interview, "I do not believe we want to tell people they can't have procedures that have a realistic chance of saving their lives and returning to normal."

Time magazine reported that Mrs. Clinton wants to "change the culture of dying" and quoted an unnamed administration official as saying, "That's why Hillary's talking up living wills and advance directives. She hopes to spur others to get comfortable with pulling the plug" (Michael Kramer, "Pulling the Plug," *Time* [4 October 1993]: 36).

Surgeon General Jocelyn Elders even weighed in with criticism of our current health care system, which she says is a system of "paying for dying," lamenting that 90 percent of spending takes place in the last few months of life. She would like to see greater spending on preventive medicine for children, spending she describes as an "investment rather than an expenditure" ("Elders Again Calls for Drug-Legalization Study," [15 January 1994]: A3). The discussion of human life in terms of investments and expenditures demonstrates just how far this nation has travelled from belief in the sanctity of human life. When euthanasia first reared its ugly head, the pro life movement warned that the "right to die" would become the "duty to die." As Burke Balch of the National Right to Life Committee (NRLC) aptly stated, "Rationing based on quality of life is just another name for selective involuntary euthanasia, euthanasia that discriminates on the basis of age and disability."

The comments coming out of the Clinton administration should serve as a warning that cost-effectiveness will become the determining factor in decisions regarding access to medical care. Even relatively inexpensive services may be denied if providers determine that the person's "quality of life" will be such that they are not worth saving when measured against the risk of the alliance exceeding its budget.

4. Who will do the rationing?

The federal government will set the limits, but alliance officials and health plans will do the rationing. This legislation is designed to make fee-for-service plans obsolete and push people into managed care plans that already have procedures in place to restrain cost by rationing care. As Elizabeth McCaughey points out in a *Wall Street Journal* article, "HMOs have a track record of tightly controlling the use of tests and expensive drugs, limiting patient access to doctors through gatekeepers, restricting patient choice of pharmacies and hospitals, and penalizing patients who get emergency care outside the HMO network."[5]

5. What do economists have to say about the price controls in the plan?

Five hundred and sixty-five economists wrote a letter to President Clinton on 13 January 1994 urging him to exclude price controls, in any form, from the plan. They reminded the president of the "social and economic disaster" of price controls on gasoline in the 1970s. They also pointed out that we have four thousand years of universal experience with governments trying to hold down prices by regulation and need only to look at history to see that these regulations did nothing but cause "shortages, black markets and reduced quality."

These economists, some even avid Clinton supporters, concluded, "Caps, fee schedules and other government regulations may appear to reduce medical spending, but such gains are illusory. We will instead end up with lower-quality medical care, reduced medical innovation, and expensive new bureaucracies to monitor compliance. These controls will hurt people and they will damage the economy."

6. How will the Clinton proposal and its controls affect research and development of new treatments?

While government grants are provided for in the legislation, the controls of the act could discourage private investment in research and development. Lisa Raines, vice president of a biotechnology company called Genzyme Corporation stated that Clinton's controls "would be devastating to the ability of companies to raise the capital needed to develop breakthrough drugs for Alzheimer's disease and other unmet medical needs."[6]

7. How will the disabled be affected by this legislation?

Any discussion of the Clinton proposal and its effects upon the disabled should begin with discussion of the inherently discriminatory provisions. One provision states that unless it is intentional, discrimination on the basis of "business necessity" is not prohibited.[7] While this provision does not specifically target the disabled or the elderly, both groups should be aware that a loophole of this nature exists.

With regard to the disabled, the legislation states that outpatient occupational therapy, physical therapy, and speech therapy include "only items or services used to restore functional capacity or minimize limitations on physical and cognitive functions as a result of an illness or injury."[8] In other words, congenital abnormalities are not covered under this provision. Even the bill's definition of a rehabilitation facility includes the fact that this facility is for "rehabilitation from illness or injury."

Children born with disabilities that require rehabilitation to increase function may be denied under this act. Randall O'Donnell, president of Kansas City, Missouri, Children's Mercy Hospital testified that the act will not "cover the needs of the child with a chronic or congenital condition, such as cerebral palsy."[9] Clinton administration officials acknowledge that the act would deny therapy to children with "cerebral palsy, cystic fibrosis and other congenital and chronic disabilities" because such treatment is considered too costly.[10]

Even the cases of those disabled as the result of an illness or injury will be subject to review after sixty days to determine whether rehabilitation should continue. The treatment can only be continued if the reviewer determines that "functioning is improving."[11] Disabled Americans who need treatment to maintain a certain level of function may be denied treatment after sixty days under this provision. The most pathetic aspect of this legislation with regard to the disabled is that the act would pay for prenatal diagnosis of disabilities and abortion to end the lives of babies, but it would not pay for therapy for these same children. In essence, parents of an unborn child with a disability are given a financial incentive to abort.

Across this country, the lives of the

disabled become increasingly more un-
certain as debates rage on regarding the
denial of treatment. National Right to
Life Committee vice president Robert
Powell, a paraplegic, asserted, "We—
people with disabilities—are the only
group of human beings who have to justify our very existence" (Robert Powell,
"Clinton's Health Care Rationing Plan
Threatens the Disabled," *NRL News* [7
December 1993]: 3). Passage of this legislation, given the above provisions and
the Clintons' "quality of life" criteria,
would effectively end the debate and
serve as a disgusting commentary on the
low value this nation places on the lives
of disabled Americans.

8. Are the elderly in jeopardy given the fact that rationing of medical care will occur?

Many questions arise concerning the
"appropriateness" of medical procedures
for the elderly in the face of dwindling
budgets. Will it be appropriate for the
elderly to receive expensive medical treatments when they are no longer contrib-
uting to the economic well-being of the
nation? In a nation concerned more with
cost-effectiveness than human life, will

care for the elderly be considered a "good investment"? Reports coming out of countries that have socialized medicine do not bode well for our older Americans. Nation after nation reports that the elderly are routinely denied necessary medical treatment or placed on waiting lists behind younger patients considered a better investment.

If the Clinton proposal passes at a time when our baby boomers approach the age that they place a greater strain on the nation's limited health care budget, the elderly will, in all likelihood, learn very quickly that insurance coverage does not necessarily guarantee access.

5 | Socialized Medicine Equals Health (In) Security

As the health care debate rages on, much attention has been focused on the systems of other countries. If the Clinton proposal is indeed socialized medicine, it is only natural for the American public to be curious about what our future would look like based upon countries who already live under a similar system.

Canada and its system of national health insurance is a fine example of the problems found in any system of socialized medicine. Despite reports coming out of Canada with details on the rationing of services and waiting lists, the drafters of the Health Security Act adopted our northern neighbor's system of global budgets and price controls. Canada as well as the systems of socialized medi-

cine in other nations offer America a
glimpse of her future under the Health
(In) Security Act.

1. What is socialized medicine?

According to *Mosby's Medical and Nursing Dictionary*, socialized medicine is "a
system of delivery of health care in which
the expense of care is borne by a governmental agency supported by taxation
rather than being paid for directly by the
client on a fee-for-service or contract
basis."

2. Is the Clinton proposal socialized medicine?

Yes. This legislation would put our
entire health care system under the control of the federal government with states
and regional alliances in the role of enforcing federal policy. The program is to
be largely paid for by employer mandated
coverage which the Congressional Budget Office insists is a tax on business,
much to the chagrin of the Clintons who
wanted to avoid calling it a tax.

3. Does the Health Security Act pro-
pose a system similar to the Canadian system?

Without going into great detail about the delivery of health care services in Canada and how the system operates, it is sufficient to say that the Canadian system is socialized medicine and that some of the most significant problem areas of the system are replicated in the Clinton proposal. The areas on which this handbook will concentrate are governmental control, global budgeting, and price controls.

All ten of the Canadian provinces and two territories operate similar, but not identical, single-payer systems in which each province administers and finances its own universal health plan. Government regulation, global budgeting, and price controls are an integral part of the administration of health care in Canada. After all, what the government pays for, it has the right to regulate!

4. Much attention has been given to the details of the Clinton proposal, but what are the general effects of complete government control over one-seventh of our economy?

First and foremost, individual freedoms are abridged. No longer do individuals have any choices or input on a variety of different questions regarding their health care. Employers and employees are robbed of the opportunity to decide health benefits in employment negotiations. Individuals are coerced by law into paying for a percentage of health insurance they may not desire. Regulation compromises the ability of doctors to choose treatments that are in the best interest of their patients.

Socialized medicine is incompatible with the perpetuation of individual freedoms. We cannot accept government control over one aspect of our lives without jeopardizing our freedoms in every other sphere. The basic premise underlying socialism is that individuals have lost the ability to manage themselves so they must be managed by external controls. If we adopt this premise in health care, it is only a question of time before the premise manages us.

The second serious consequence is that government control undermines individual responsibility. In assessing the inevitable failure of socialized medicine in Canada, one columnist wrote,

> The basic problem with Canada's system is that it imposes no respon-

sibility on either users or providers of services to be prudent in their use of facilities and services. Totally open-ended and gold-plated, our medical system is wasteful and is destined, this decade, to result in wholesale rationing of services and cancerous cost increases due to our aging population. The system is inefficient because there is no competition, nor are there any built-in incentives to save money while achieving results. (Diane Francis, "Expensive and Dangerous Myths," *Maclean's* [2 September 1991]: 13)

This columnist's point is well taken. External regulations cannot replace or provide any efficient substitute for the responsible choices of individuals. A nation that robs its people of the opportunity to exercise responsibility in any sphere will ultimately beget a people who need and expect to be governed.

The third outgrowth of government control is the destruction of the medical profession. Damage is first inflicted upon the public's perception of the vocation in an effort to sell centralized control. As Dr. Anna Scherzer explains, the sales pitch goes something like: "Those rich doctors are getting richer from your sorrows and miseries. Mr. and Mrs. Average America, you deserve better. . . . Don't worry. You'll only have to make small sacrifices so that you and your children have the future you deserve. . . . Of course, to get these benefits and make them equitable, there will have to be protocols, standards, supervision . . ."[1] If skeptical about whether Dr. Scherzer's sales pitch is accurate, review the rhetoric of the Clinton campaign.

Once government control is reality, physicians lose the right to be independent practitioners. They are no longer permitted to practice their craft according to their conscience. The physician's role is to serve the political and fiscal goals of the state.

The fourth ramification is that a nation's most vulnerable populations are viewed as a liability. Precious resources are begrudged those who are sick or impaired. The elderly who no longer contribute to the work force are regarded as nothing more than a drain on the economy.

In Germany after World War I, the concept *lebensunwertes Leben* was adopted. In translation, it means, "life not worthy of life itself."[2] Certain life, weighed against the limited resources of that time, was not to be sustained.

The Clinton plan with its "medically necessary" and "appropriate" language is not so very different. Will certain life be judged "not worthy of medical treatment" under Mrs. Clinton's quality of life ethic? Will our nation begin to weigh human life in terms of investments and expenditures? We have only to look at the medical decisions made every day in other nations subsisting under the heavy hand of government control to see our future.

Finally, privacy is no longer respected. Intricate information networks designed to monitor compliance give the specifics of every case. Confidentiality within the doctor-patient relationship, once thought to be sacrosanct, is completely sabotaged. Take a look at the Information Network outlined in the Clinton legislation.

5. What are the effects of global budgeting and price controls in Canada?

There are many. In the interest of space, we will concentrate on a few significant effects. First, we have only to look at Canada to see that government regulation of budgets through price controls will lead to the rationing of services. Canadians can see a primary care physician with little trouble, but moving beyond primary care to see a specialist is difficult.

The Fraser Institute in Vancouver, British Columbia, explains that "the Canadian system responds to excess demand by making people get in line for medical treatment."[3] An estimated 1,379,000 have their names on lists waiting for some type of medical service.[4] Another 177 thousand are waiting for some type of service and 45 percent say that they are "in pain" while they wait.[5] The number of operations performed in Canada between 1986 and 1989 decreased by 4 percent while waiting lists grew.[6]

The average wait among the provinces to see a specialist is five weeks. After seeing a specialist, there is frequently another waiting list for the time between the specialist's recommendation for treatment and the delivery of that treatment. The total waiting time between being referred by a general practitioner to receiving treatment ranges from eleven and a half weeks in Ontario to twenty-one weeks on Prince Edward Island. Across the nation, patients wait for coronary bypass surgery while the Canadian press reports of patients dying on the waiting lists.[7]

When people boast about the Canadian system controlling costs better than the United States, the implication is that they are able to hold down costs while delivering adequate medical care as demand rises. However, upon closer examination, we find quite a different scenario. The Canadian system does not offer more medical care as demand rises. It holds down costs by limiting government spending on health care and when demand exceeds the budget, it puts people on waiting lists. Meanwhile, many hospitals run at less than full capacity because provinces do not have the money to pay for their services.

Another form of rationing is the limiting of access to technology. The United States has ten times as many magnetic resonance imaging (MRI) units per capita as Canada. We have three times as many lithotripsy units as Canada, and Canadians wait six weeks to receive lithotripsy while the average Washingtonian can get it in roughly three weeks. The United States has three times as many computerized axial tomography (CAT) scanners per person. And per capita, our nation has three times as many open-heart surgery units and eleven times as many cardiac catheterization units as our neighbor to the north.[8] According to Dr. Robert MacMillan, minister of health insurance for the Ontario Ministry of Health, "All of Canada faces a lag in accessibility, particularly in highly sophisticated care."[9]

Dr. MacMillan says that referring patients to the United States for care serves as a "safety valve" for a system that is overwhelmed. In May 1993, Ontario signed contracts with U.S. hospitals for acquired brain injury care. They were also considering contracts for "child and adolescent psychiatric, eating disorder, and drug and alcohol addiction treatment. Canadians now account for 75 percent of the patients in the chemical dependency unit at Falls Memorial Hospital, International Falls, Minnesota."[10]

A study reported in the *New England Journal of Medicine* indicated that roughly one-third of Canadian physicians referred patients outside their country for treatment in the last five years. That figure should be compared with 7 percent in the United States. About 10 percent of all British Columbia residents needing cancer therapy have been sent to the United States.[11] Canadians make up almost half of the in vitro fertilization patients at the University of Washington Medical Center. These patients pay about five thousand dollars out-of-pocket for each procedure.[12] The Ontario Health Insurance Plan paid nearly $214 million to U.S. physicians and hospitals in 1990.[13]

Bureaucratic delays caused by large amounts of paper work and lengthy approval procedures compromise treatment. In 1992, the Canadian Hemophilia Society reported that bureaucratic delays in implementing blood screening rules based on heat treatment resulted in eight hundred of Canada's two thousand hemophiliacs being infected with the HIV virus in 1985.[14] These same delays could occur under the Health Security Act, particularly with breakthrough drugs where the National Health Board and an Advisory Council evaluate the prices of new drugs based on a host of criteria.

Because there are no national waiting lists, inequities in the length of time patients wait are inevitable. The NCPA finds that global budgets discriminate against the elderly, the poor, racial minorities, and rural patients. Among the elderly, the United States performs twice as many coronary artery bypass operations on the elderly per capita as Canada does. With those seventy-five and older, the difference between the countries is four to one.[15]

The probability of waiting on lists for treatment is much less for high-income groups than for low to middle-income groups. Higher income groups are more knowledgeable about maneuvering through the sea of bureaucratic red tape.

NCPA found that "Canada's principal minority group—Indians—fares less well than American Indians."[16]

Rural patients are also discriminated against given the fact that restricted funding results in specialists and modern technology being located in major cities.

The final form of rationing is in the quality of care. Budget constraints tend to result in physicians providing only minimal care, and the principal way to control cost is by denying care altogether. One report indicated that 25 percent of all acute-care hospital beds are occupied by chronically ill patients who use the hospitals as nursing homes. New Brunswick's Moncton Hospital kept patients in hallways and even closets while twenty three hundred other people sat on waiting lists.[17]

Another practice is "bed-blocking" in which chronically ill patients are left in beds to block admission of patients with more costly illnesses—all with hospital administrators consent. This is one type of perverse incentives that price constraints inspire.

6. Does the Canadian system control costs?

No. Despite rhetoric to the contrary, Canada has done no better job in controlling costs even with the rationing of services and the deterioration in the quality of care. From 1967 to 1987, studies show that real increases in per capita spending on health care were virtually the same with Canada's increase of 4.58 percent just slightly higher than the United States' 4.38 percent increase.[18]

7. What other nations can we look to for examples of the negative consequences of socialized medicine?

A Canadian columnist wrote,

> In a planned Utopia, every bit of autonomy—financial or otherwise—

that an individual might have in a free enterprise society takes second place to the requirements of the social engineers running the place. The only hope that citizens may have is that they will run things well. The reality is that they often run them poorly, but in any case they run them. (Barbara Amiel, "State Coercion: A Case History," *Maclean's* [24 May 1993]: 9.)

Although this columnist is from Canada, the same situation is true in any nation that has tried the planned utopia of socialized medicine. Great Britain has a population of 55 million and 800 thousand sit on waiting lists for surgery. One out of every four beds sits empty in Britain because the National Health Service (NHS) cannot pay hospitals.[19]

Rationing of care has caused many in Great Britain to seek private insurance. In fact, Dr. Eamonn Butler of the Adam Smith Institute in London, wrote,

Policy analysts in the United Kingdom derive wry amusement from the fact that America seems determined to model its health care system on what we, in the UK, are trying to get away from. . . . British citizens are leaving the NHS in droves just at the time when U.S. policy makers seemed determined to re-create it in America. (Eamonn Butler, "The National Health Service in the United Kingdom: Model for the United States?" *The Journal of the Medical Association of Georgia* [December 1993]: 643–5.)

In New Zealand fifty thousand of its three million people are waiting for surgery and one out of every five beds stands empty.[20]

Sweden presents much the same picture. Health policy analyst Edmund Haislmaier stated, "In Sweden, a low birthweight baby weighing less than a certain amount would bring an immediate decision. . . . The doctor would come to the mother and say: 'I'm sorry, this baby is too premature and can't live.' The decision is already made."[21]

6 | Alternative Proposals

With debate focused on the Health Security Act, many fail to realize that there are alternatives to the Clintons' proposal for socialized medicine. Some combination of these acts is likely to pass, but there is only one proposal that remains true to the principles of a free market economy. It will probably not go anywhere, but as one columnist wrote, "At least it is intellectually honest."

1. Are there any alternatives to the Clinton Health Security Act?

Yes. Numerous plans have been introduced in Congress to address the problems with our health care system. Over on the left side of the spectrum with the Clinton plan is legislation introduced by

Representative Jim McDermott (D-WA), which would establish a single-payer system, much like the Canadian system. McDermott's proposal would include abortion as "medically necessary elective surgery."

Another that is just to the right of the Health Security Act is the Managed Competition Act of 1993 introduced by Representatives Jim Cooper (D-TN) and Fred Grandy (R-IA). It provides for a national health board and purchasing cooperatives with exclusive territories. The national health board would determine the benefit package, and the plan would mandate participation by self-employed individuals and small employers. The Cooper/Grandy bill offers the opportunity to create (Medical Savings Accounts) MSAs.

Two proposals lie in the center of the political spectrum, each offering some form of managed competition. A proposal by Senator John Chafee (R-RI), dubbed the official "Republican" alternative, would mandate that all individuals buy their own insurance, and employers merely provide the opportunity. An independent commission would establish a minimum benefit package, and premiums would be decided on the basis of "community rating."

Senator Don Nickles (R-OK) and Representative Cliff Stearns (R-FL) introduced a proposal that would require individuals to buy health insurance or face tax penalties and calls for modified "community rating." Both the Chafee and Nickles/Stearns bills offer MSAs (explained in detail later).

None of the three more moderate alternatives create the bureaucracy of the Clinton plan, and all offer tax relief to those who purchase their own health insurance, but not one of them promotes the principles of a free market economy like the proposal introduced by Senator Phil Gramm (R-TX). The Gramm proposal, the "Comprehensive Family Health Access and Savings Act," would require employers to offer three health plan options including an HMO option, but the linchpin of his proposal is the MSA. MSAs empower individuals to make responsible health care choices rather than empowering government to establish external regulations. These MSAs are tax-free personal accounts used to pay medical expenses that are not covered by insurance. People could confine their insurance to catastrophic coverage and reduce their premium payments. The savings in premiums could be deposited in the MSAs. Deposits could be made by employers and employees, but they would be the property of individuals. Employers would deposit the money they previously paid in insurance premiums for the employee.

Each holder of an MSA could withdraw money without penalty, and money that was not used could continue to accrue interest. Upon retirement, a person could roll the money over into an IRA or private pension plan.

Unlike Clinton's bureaucratic command-and-control system, MSAs would encourage people to be prudent in their health care choices. With third parties paying the bills, there is no incentive for the patient or the doctor to think about cost. Using MSAs to pay medical expenses would encourage patients to scrutinize medical bills like they do other bills. Physicians would be encouraged to exercise more restraint in their fees and the number of procedures they perform. These accounts would give people back the control over their health that many HMOs have undermined and the Clinton proposal would rob them of altogether. Both individual freedom and responsibility are encouraged through these MSAs, and the market is allowed to operate freely and control cost.

With patients empowered, the doctor-patient relationship could remain intact. Patients could stay with the doctors with whom they are comfortable, and doctors could treat patients in accordance with their best medical knowledge. Privacy also is protected because there is no need for monitoring by bureaucrats.

People would not be required to carry insurance, but MSAs would encourage people to acquire it. Many more individuals would be willing to pay into an account that they could roll over into an IRA or pension plan than they would to pay for insurance they may never use.

In yet another effort to control health care costs, the Gramm bill offers meaningful medical liability reform. It enacts a statute of limitations of two years in most cases and no more than four years in cases with extenuating circumstances. It caps noneconomic damages at two hundred fifty thousand dollars and in economic damages, no more than one hundred thousand dollars can be required in a lump sum. For amounts over one hundred thousand dollars, the defendant shall be permitted to make periodic payments at intervals determined by the court. Attorneys fees are limited to 25 percent of the first one hundred fifty thousand dollars recovered and 15 percent of any amount in excess of the first one hundred fifty thousand dollars.[1]

7 | Conclusion

Drafters of the Health Security Act claim that it will restore six fundamental principles to our health care system. These principles are security, simplicity, savings, choice, quality, and individual responsibility. However, when measured against its own standards, the Health Security Act is an utter failure.

There is no security in legislation that advances the killing of the unborn, introduces price controls which will lead to rationing and waiting lists, and espouses subjective "quality of life" and cost-benefit ratios in determining "medically necessary" and/or "appropriate" treatment.

Simplicity cannot be achieved in a system designed to micromanage health care delivery. Patients and physicians will swim in a sea of paperwork, and only those skilled at maneuvering through bureaucratic red tape will receive the treatment they need.

Savings cannot be generated by legislation that expands the size of the federal government by 20 percent and increases the national deficit by $74 billion while offering an expensive, one-size-fits-all benefit package. On the contrary, what we can expect is a sharp increase in our taxes to finance this entitlement nightmare.

Quality in health care delivery is a reality in America. We have the highest cure rates for many forms of cancer and are unmatched in our treatment of heart disease. This legislation, through its global budgets and price controls, will wage war on the quality health care workers have strived so hard to achieve.

Finally, legislation that robs individuals of the opportunity to make even the smallest of decisions regarding their health care needs cannot promote responsibility. If anything, this act will breed a people who need and expect to be cared for and managed.

Our president is too bright an individual to believe for a moment that this legislation promotes any of the six principles we hear him recite time and again. While they make for nice rhetoric, the sad truth is that they are nothing more than part of a deceptive marketing campaign by the Clinton administration.

Americans cannot afford to ignore this debate. We must ask questions of our legislators and require honest answers. If the Clinton proposal passes, it will serve as a "foot in the door" for those who would like to see our nation become a socialist state. This is not alarmist rhetoric; it is truth.

When evaluating the various proposals now before Congress, keep in mind that there is no "utopia" somewhere between a free market and socialism. Health security can only be achieved as people, not government, are empowered to make responsible choices regarding their consumption of medical services. Settling for a system that achieves anything less would mean that the American people had fallen prey to the Clinton facade.

Notes

Chapter One

1. "The Myth of Universal Coverage," The National Center for Policy Analysis (NCPA) (14 February 1993).

2. Ibid.

3. Ibid.

4. Health Security Act, Title I, Subtitle D, Section 1345(d)(2).

5. William J. Baumol, "Do Health Care Costs Matter?" *The New Republic* (22 November 1993): 16–8.

6. Ibid., 18 .

7. Robert J. Samuelson, "Health Care: How We Got Into This Mess," *Newsweek* (4 October 1993): 31.

Chapter Two

1. Health Security Act, Title I, Subtitle F, Section 1505(e).

2. Health Security Act, Title I, Subtitle B, Section 1141(a)(1).

3. Health Security Act, Title I, Subtitle C, Section 1154.

4. Health Security Act, Title I, Subtitle D, Section 1323(i)(2).

5. Health Security Act, Title I, Subtitle C, Section 1202(b)(3).

6. Health Security Act, Title I, Subtitle C, Section 1223.

7. Health Security Act, Title I, Subtitle C, Section 1222.

8. Health Security Act, Title I, Subtitle D, Section 1321.

9. Health Security Act, Title I, Subtitle D, Section 1322.

10. Health Security Act, Title I, Subtitle D, Section 1322.

11. Elizabeth McCaughey, "No Exit: What the Clinton Plan Will Do for You," *The New Republic* (7 February 1994): 21–5.

12. Health Security Act, Title I, Subtitle D, Section 1385.

13. Health Security Act, Title VII, Subtitle A, Section 7121.

14. Health Security Act, Title I, Subtitle D, Section 1397.

15. John C. Goodman and Gerald L. Musgrave, "A Primer on Managed Competition," The National Center for Policy Analysis (NCPA) (1 March 1994): Draft 21.

16. Ibid.

17. Ibid.

18. Health Security Act, Title I, Subtitle E, Section 1422.

19. Health Security Act, Title I, Subtitle E, Section 1003.

20. Health Security Act, Title IV, Subtitle A, Section 4001.

21. Health Security Act, Title IV, Subtitle B, Section(s) 4101–4106.

22. Health Security Act, Title II, Subtitle A, Section 2001.

23. Health Security Act, Title II, Subtitle A, Section 2003.

24. Robert E. Moffett, "A Guide to the Clinton Health Plan," *Heritage Talking Points* (19 November 1993): 31.

25. Daniel J. Mitchell, "The Economic and Budget Impact of the Clinton Health Plan," *Heritage Backgrounder* (13 January 1994): 6.

26. Karen Riley and J. Jennings Moss, "Health Numbers Disputed," *The Washington Times* (9 February 1994).

27. Ibid.

28. Moffett, "A Guide to the Clinton Plan," 26.

29. Health Security Act, Title III, Subtitle A, Section 3011.

Chapter Three

1. Health Security Act, Title I, Subtitle B, Section 1116.

2. Douglas Johnson, "Clintons Push Plan To Multiply Abortion Access, While Telling the Public They Seek 'No Change,' " *NRL News* (30 September 1993): 1.

3. "Pro-Abortion Groups Pressure Congress for Clinton Bill to Make Abortion A Federal Mandate," *NRL News* (3 February 1994): 1.

4. Douglas Johnson, "Clintons Push Plan to Multiply Abortion Access, While Telling the Public They Seek 'No Change,' " *NRL News* (30 September 1993): 1.

5. Ibid.

6. Ibid.

7. Ibid.

8. Health Security Act, Title I, Subtitle C, Section 1162.

9. Health Security Act, Title III, Subtitle G, Section(s) 3861-3862.

10. Health Security Act, Title III, Subtitle G, Section 3863.

11. Health Security Act, Title I, Subtitle F, Section 1582.

12. Health Security Act, Title III, Subtitle G, Section 3601.

13. Health Security Act, Title III, Subtitle G, Section 3602.

Chapter Four

1. Robert E. Moffett, "A Guide to the Clinton Health Plan," *Heritage Talking Points* (19 November 1993): 33.

2. Health Security Act, Title V, Subtitle C, Section 5201(e)(3).

3. Health Security Act, Title V, Subtitle E, Section 5434.

4. William J. Baumol, "Do Health Care Costs Matter?" *The New Republic* (22 November 1993): 16–8.

5. Elizabeth McCaughey, "Clinton Plan=Price Controls," *NRL News* (7 December 1993): 10.

6. Burke J. Balch, "Research and Development of Lifesaving Treatments: The Impact of the Clinton Rationing Plan," *NRL News* (30 September 1993): 9.

7. Health Security Act, Title I, Subtitle E, Section 1402(c)(3).

8. Health Security Act, Title I, Subtitle B, Section 1123(b)(1).

9. Burke J. Balch, "Save Lives of Those Who Will 'Return to Normal' Clinton Says," *NRL News* (7 December 1993): 1.

10. Burke Balch, "First Lady Tells Congress Quality of Life Basis for Rationing," *NRL News* (19 October 1993): 1.

11. Health Security Act, Title I, Subtitle B, Section 1123(b)(2).

Chapter Five

1. Dr. Anna Scherzer, "The Holocaust Museum: Lessons for American Medicine," Association of American Physicians and Surgeons Annual Meeting (8 October 1993).

2. Ibid.

3. David Boaz, "Canada Offers Faulty Model," *Insight* (13 September 1993): 30.

4. Michael Walker and John C. Goodman, "What President Clinton Can Learn from Canada About Price Controls and Global Budgets," *NCPA Policy Backgrounder* (5 October 1993): 2.

5. Ibid.

6. Boaz, "Canada Offers Faulty Model," 30.

7. Walker and Goodman, "What President Clinton Can Learn," 6.

8. Ibid., 2.

9. Marcia Berss, "Our System Is Just Overwhelmed," *Forbes* (24 May 1993): 40.

10. Ibid.

11. Boaz, "Canada Offers Faulty Model," 30.

12. Walker and Goodman, "What President Clinton Can Learn," 9.

13. Ibid.

14. "Hemophiliacs Say Bureaucratic Delays Lead To HIV Infections," *AIDS Weekly* (16 November 1992): 11.

15. Walker and Goodman, "What President Clinton Can Learn," 11.

16. Ibid.

17. Ibid., 14.

18. Ibid., 15.

19. "Debate Rages Over Canadian Health Care System," *National Underwriter Life and Health-Financial Services* (3 December 1990): 31.

20. Ibid.

21. Burke J. Balch, "Rationing, Euthanasia, and the Clinton Health Plan," *NRL News* (14 September 1993): 1.

Chapter Six

1. The Comprehensive Family Health Access and Savings Act.

More Good Books from Huntington House

Gays & Guns
The Case against Homosexuals in the Military
by John Eidsmoe, Ph.D.

The homosexual revolution seeks to overthrow the Laws of Nature. A Lieutenant Colonel in the United States Air Force Reserve, Dr. John Eidsmoe eloquently contends that admitting gays into the military would weaken the combat effectiveness of our armed forces. This cataclysmic step would also legitimize homosexuality, a lifestyle that most Americans know is wrong.

While echoing Cicero's assertion that "a sense of what is right is common to all mankind," Eidsmoe rationally defends his belief. There are laws that govern the universe, he reminds us. Laws that compel the earth to rotate on its axis, laws that govern the economy; and so there is also a moral law that governs man's nature. The violation of this moral law is physically, emotionally and spiritually destructive. It is destructive to both the individual and to the community of which he is a member.

ISBN Trade Paper 1-56384-043-X $7.99
ISBN Hardcover 1-56384-046-4 $14.99

Kinsey, Sex and Fraud:
The Indoctrination of a People
by Dr. Judith A. Reisman and
Edward Eichel

Kinsey, Sex and Fraud describes the research of Alfred Kinsey which shaped Western society's beliefs and understanding of the nature of human sexuality. His unchallenged conclusions are taught at every level of education—elementary, high school, and college—and quoted in textbooks as undisputed truth.

The authors clearly demonstrate that Kinsey's research involved illegal experimentations on several hundred children. The survey was carried out on a non-representative group of Americans, including disproportionately large numbers of sex offenders, prostitutes, prison inmates, and exhibitionists.

ISBN 0-910311-20-X $10.99

Homeless in America:
The Solution
by Jeremy Reynalds

Author Jeremy Reynald's current shelter, Joy Junction, located in Albuquerque, New Mexico, has become the state's largest homeless shelter. Beginning with fifty dollars in his pocket and a lot of compassion, Jeremy Reynalds now runs a shelter that has a yearly budget of over $600,000. He receives no government or United Way funding. Anyone who desires to help can, says Reynalds.

ISBN 1-56384-063-4 $9.99

Political Correctness: The Cloning of the American Mind
by David Thibodaux, Ph.D.

The author, a professor of literature at the University of Southwestern Louisiana, confronts head on the movement that is now being called Political Correctness. Political correctness, says Thibodaux, "is an umbrella under which advocates of civil rights, gay and lesbian rights, feminism, and environmental causes have gathered." To express traditionally Western concepts in universities today can result in not only ostracism, but even suspension. (According to a recent "McNeil-Lehrer News Hour" report, one student was suspended for discussing the reality of the moral law with an avowed homosexual. He was reinstated only after he apologized.)

ISBN 1-56384-026-X Trade Paper $9.99

Conservative, American, & Jewish
by Jacob Neusner

Neusner has fought on the front lines of the culture war and here writes reports about sectors of the battles. He has taken a consistent, conservative position in the academy, federal agencies in the humanities and the arts, and in the world of religion in general and Judaism in particular. These essays set out to change minds and end up touching the hearts and souls of their readers.

ISBN 1-56384-048-0 $9.99

ORDER THESE HUNTINGTON HOUSE BOOKS !